Poisoned at the Restaurant

What Restaurants Really Feed You and How to Take One Meal Back

Marko Vovk

Copyright

This publication is intended to provide accurate and authoritative information on the subject matter covered. It is sold with the understanding that the author and publisher are not providing legal or medical advice. Readers should consult qualified professionals regarding their own situations.

For permission requests, visit: FixYourToxicHome.com.

Paperback ISBN: 978-1-969955-90-7 Ebook ISBN: 978-1-969955-28-0

Cover design: Marko Vovk (Draft 1, 2026) Interior design: Marko Vovk

Editing and production tools: Word, Book Brush, Autocrit, Grammarly Plus, Perplexity.
Review support: Friends and readers from Facebook and YouTube (channels under "Marko Vovk" and "Cleveland-Marko"). Some images created or enhanced with AI tools.

Final editing: Marko Vovk (some minor inconsistencies may remain due to no paid outside editing).
Printed in the United States of America. Portions of this material are adapted from *Poisoned at the Grocery Store: Why Shopping Fresh Is Not Enough to Escape a Toxic Food Supply* by Marko Vovk.

Author's Note

AUTHOR'S NOTE

I wrote this book as someone who has lived inside the problem, not as a distant expert. For years, I worked long inspection days and fed myself from drive-through windows, buffets, and takeout bags. The price showed up in my big toe first, then in my knees, my sleep, my blood work, and my mood. I did not want to believe my "reward" food was quietly sanding down my joints and fogging my mind, but my body kept trying to tell me.

Earlier, I wrote a book about what hides in boxes and cans at the store. This book walks into the other half of the story: the second kitchen of restaurants, buffets, cafeterias, and machines that now feed so many of our meals. I have spent years crawling through buildings, watching how people actually eat, and reading what researchers have found about ultra-processed food and long-term disease. I am not your doctor. I am a working person who finally got tired of limping through life and went looking for better answers.

What you will find in these pages is a mix of lived experience, simple science, and practical experiments. You will not find perfect plans or food-purity rules. I do not live on a mountaintop or grow every calorie I eat. I still make mistakes. I still eat out. The change is that I now see the pattern more clearly and take more meals back into my own hands.

This book is here to help you see the pattern in your own life. It will show you what hides behind menus, trays, and vending slots, and then invite you to try one small, realistic shift at a time. You will hear my story, but the most important story will be your own: what happens to your knees, sleep, sugar, and mood when you treat food as information rather than background noise.

I hope you will read this not as a new food Bible, but as a field guide and a conversation starter between you and your own body. You do not have to fix everything at once. You only have to be willing to take one meal back, listen for the response, and decide what to do next.

My Authorship

I began writing books in 2019, after Covid hurt the home-inspection business I had worked in for over forty years. Most of what I write grows out of that life: homes, health, everyday environments, and plain common sense with a focus on logic, not trends. I include bibliographies in most books so readers can see the research and related sources that support the stories and ideas.

My earlier books took a long time to finish and were not edited as deeply as I would have liked. Like any craft, writing gets better with practice, and each project has taught me how to be clearer and more helpful on the page. Some of my publications are listed in the back of this book under "Further Reading," for readers who want to explore more.

In a world flooded with new books every day, finding readers is harder, and honest, positive reviews matter more than ever. From time to time, I offer my books for free for a few days, simply to get them into more hands. If cost is a real barrier and you still want to read this work, you can reach out to me, and I will do my best to share a PDF copy.

— Marko Vovk

Disclaimer

This book is for informational and educational purposes only. It does not provide medical, nutritional, or legal advice, and it is not a substitute for professional care. Always talk with your doctor, nurse practitioner, or other qualified health care provider before making significant changes to your diet, starting or stopping medications, or deciding on treatment for any medical condition.

If you have existing diagnoses such as diabetes, heart disease, arthritis, gout, high blood pressure, kidney disease, or any other chronic illness, it is especially important to work with your care team when adjusting meals, medications, or activity.

If you think you may be having a medical emergency, call your local emergency number or seek immediate medical help. Never delay or ignore professional advice because of something you read in this book.

The stories and examples on these pages describe my experience and the experiences of others. They are not promises or guarantees of any specific result for you. Your body, your history, and your circumstances are your own. Use this book as one source of ideas and questions, alongside the guidance of qualified professionals and your own careful attention to how you feel.

Contents

Chapter One

The Toe That Tried to Warn Me

SLIDING INTO THE BOOTH with my kids after a long inspection day felt like crashing into a soft vinyl shore. Menus flashed with glossy close-ups and bright ink. Breading glistened, cheese stretched, and tall sodas sweated under the lights. The routine ran itself. Fried starter, large entree, sugar in a cup, and dessert if the kids tilted their faces just right.

Plates landed with a clatter that cut through the hum of televisions and ice. Heat, salt, and fryer fat rose in a wave that smelled like comfort and exhaustion mixed. Fries, nuggets, and macaroni got poked, rearranged, and abandoned as attention drifted to the claw machine by the restroom. My plate emptied, then theirs, because an old script in my head said wasting food was worse than grinding down joints.

On solo drives home from inspections, a glowing sign could pull my car into a drive-through lane almost without my permission. Two fish sandwiches and a coffee traded hands in seconds, a prize for crawling through basements and attics. The paper bag dropped onto a soft pile of cups and wrappers on the back floor. A heavy stomach and a quiet mind felt like proof the deal was worth it.

Then one morning, a throbbing big toe ripped the day open before the alarm could try. The joint looked like someone had screwed a hot red bulb under the skin; even the weight of a sheet felt like a hammer. My mind reached for the kindest story. Maybe I caught it on the bed frame, perhaps I stepped wrong, anything but the obvious drive-through windows and paper bags.

The pain eased after a few hours and slid into the "weird but harmless" drawer. Weeks later, the same toe flared again, pulsing with the same stubborn throb. I tried different shoes, careful steps, and new routes down the stairs. The drive-through stayed off the suspect list, and the quiet alarm got silenced one more time.

Over time, that angry toe refused to stay a local problem. Pain packed its bags and toured the body, stopping at knees, elbows, shoulders, and hands. Flares arrived, stayed for days, then vanished without warning, like surprise visits from a relative who never calls first. Each new ache got its own theory. Bad shoes, getting older, too many stairs, family history, anything but the pattern on the plate and in the cup holder.

Eventually, the word showed up. Gout. Gout is a form of arthritis where sharp crystals build up in a joint, often the big toe. Every step can feel like walking on broken glass. In a bad flare, you do not limp. You plan your entire day around how many times you can stand up.

What you eat and drink over many years can drive this. Heavy, salty, sweet, and greasy dishes feel like a reward when you are tired and hungry. They can also load the blood with more of the material that builds those crystals. The toe only knows what lands in the bloodstream, not what story you tell yourself.

Maybe the name "gout" doesn't fit your story, but the rhythm might sound familiar. Long days and short nights, with food scooped up wherever it waits near the road or the office. Breakfast from a drive-through window, lunch from a counter, dinner from an app brings bags to the porch. The routine persists because friends, coworkers, and neighbors seem to follow the same path.

Restaurant and takeout dishes are filling more weeks than food cooked in your own kitchen. Drive-through lanes and delivery apps turn commercial kitchens into a second home that never closes and never needs scrubbing. Pizza nights, coffee drinks, office lunches, and "I earned this" dinners blur into one long buffet. Nothing seems to change after a single combo or weekend feast, so the habit rolls on.

The bill for all of this does not arrive as one dramatic moment. Instead, small charges stack up: aching joints, extra pounds, rising blood sugar, higher blood pressure, and new prescriptions. Words like gout, diabetes, fatty liver, reflux, and arthritis appear in charts. Bottles promise relief for a monthly fee. Meanwhile, the restaurant, takeout, cafeteria, and vending machine loop remains intact because it still feels like everyday life.

If this sounds familiar, these pages follow your story as much as they trace mine. A handicap placard or a swollen toe might not yet be part of your picture. Maybe it is only fatigue, stiffness, foggy thinking, or the feeling of being much older after certain dinners. That is how this path begins, not with a crash, but with a fork.

The chapters ahead pull back the curtain on restaurant, takeout, cafeteria, and vending machine food. All of it is built from the same factory parts. Those parts were exposed in my earlier work, "Poisoned at the Grocery Store."

Cheap meats, stripped flours, seed fats, sugars, additives, dyes, and preservatives leave plants and reappear on plates without labels or warning boxes. Recipes hide behind logos, mascots, and menu names rather than ingredient panels and barcodes. Your body does not read signs. It simply has to process whatever shows up.

Together, we will walk through the restaurant ritual from the first craving to the last dirty dish. Tired, busy, lonely, or celebrating, the same doors keep swinging open. Menus, photos, and app screens nudge choices with colors, bundles, and limited-time offers. Behind the counter, unseen steps transform boxes and bags into plates and takeout containers.

Cafeterias and school lines serve children and workers a steady stream of factory products dressed up with wellness words. Machines and grab-and-go coolers keep sweet drinks, salt, and additives within reach from early morning until late at night. Step by step, this system wears down knees, guts, hearts, minds, and spirits without fireworks or sirens. Along the way, pockets of control and choice still exist, even when they seem buried.

This book will not demand a permanent break with every restaurant on your map. That would ignore real life and pretend habits built over decades can vanish in a month.

Instead, the goal is to spotlight the worst traps and the small shifts that bring the most significant returns. Changing what and how you eat can become a small rite of passage. Not a punishment, but a way to return to living in your own skin. In simple terms, this book argues that the second kitchen is quietly driving pain, fog, and chronic disease. It also argues that taking even one meal back into your own hands can begin to turn that around.

In simple terms, here is the deal this chapter is offering you:

The second kitchen of restaurants, takeout, cafeterias, and vending machines is changing your joints, blood sugar, mood, and long-term health.
Your body is already sending messages through toes, knees, energy, and foggy mornings about how that system is working out.
You don't have to give up eating out forever to change your story.
You can start by taking one meal back into your own hands and watching what happens.
The chapters ahead will show you where the harm hides and where your choices still matter most.

Chapter Two

Seeing Through the Buffet

WALKING INTO THE ALL-YOU-CAN-EAT buffet, I already know what comes next. My joints realize it, too. These days, pain does not wait for tomorrow. It moves from the toe to the ankle to the knee soon after I eat.

The sign outside promises variety and value. Rows of steel pans shine under warm lamps, steam rising like a welcome. Years ago, this place was pure excitement: endless choices, low prices, no dishes.

Now, after writing "Poisoned at the Grocery Store" and reading labels for months, I cannot stop seeing what is really on these trays. I look at the sushi and do not see art. I see crowded tanks I would not swim in and long shipping routes. I see rice from fields that may share soil with metals or old chemicals.

The fresh shine looks less like a clean ocean and more like careful hands. It seems more like treatments and glazes.

Beauty on the outside, chemistry behind the glass. The story on the tray and the story in my head no longer match.

At the hot tables, more ingredients scroll through my mind than the menu ever admits. Sweet sauces glow with sugar and thickeners. Orange glazes might as well be half syrup and half dye. Fried items carry a double load. Old seed fat in the fryer plus batter mixes read like lab notes.

In my mind, I can see flavor powders and factory starches hiding behind names like 'chef special' and 'house sauce'. Those names sound homemade. They cover bags and buckets in the back room.

The drink station at the end of the line looks like a dessert bar in liquid form. Cola, lemon-lime, bright orange, and fake-fruit teas wait in endless loops. A refill is not a little more soda. It is another shot of sugar, acid, and color poured over ice.

Watching a child go back for a fourth cup hits a nerve. Part of me wants to say this is not just a drink. The cup looks harmless. The pattern is not.

As I pick up a plate, I give myself a quiet talk. Do not be picky. Take a little rice, some chicken, a salad, and stop there. Act normal. That is what I tell myself while my body mutters, "We know how this ends."

The line moves faster than my judgment. The cold bar looks fresh, with sliced fruit, rolls, and salads. The hot bar smells like comfort, holidays, and home. By the time I reach the end, my plate looks like a greatest hits album of everything I meant to avoid.

The next morning, the limp is back. Some days it is the ankle. Some days it is the knee. Some days, fingers will not grip a pen.

Doctors called it gout once. Now I call it food pain. It is my body's running commentary on what I chose the night before. The message is not subtle.

Aching joints, stiff fingers, swollen feet, constant heartburn, headaches, foggy thinking, or an unsettled gut all fit the same pattern. Many people live a version of this story. The list of labels can grow long. Diabetes, high pressure, high cholesterol, reflux, arthritis, migraines, irritable bowel, fatty liver, asthma, or "just getting older."

Most doctors mean well, but the cycle is familiar. Each new ache or odd lab value earns a new name and a new pill. Pressure pills, metformin, statins, acid reducers, pain pills, inhalers, and sleep aids line up on counters. The prescription list keeps growing, but the menu stays the same.

Very few people hear that a lifetime of restaurant plates, takeout bags, cafeteria trays, and snacks from machines might be pouring fuel on inflammation week after week. It is easier to blame age, stress, or bad genes than to point at the plate. It feels safer to believe the body has worn out than to admit the hotline has helped grind it down.

What changed for me was not just my joints. Reading labels for the grocery store book showed that most restaurant food comes from the same system as the boxes and cans at home. The buffet is not a magical kitchen with a grandmother in the back. It is a delivery point for factories and bulk suppliers.

Ingredients arrive in bags, tubs, and frozen blocks. The labels rest on cartons in the storage room, not on the glass beside the food. Diners see shine and steam, not supply chains. The second kitchen stays hidden while the trays remain full.

Buffets are not alone. Many hot lines, salad bars, and value menus lean on ultra-processed meats, coating mixes, sauces, and blends. These items are cheap, stable, and easy to serve to crowds. The sense of variety comes from mixing and matching the same base pieces with different sauces and colors.

One tray might say sweet and sour, another orange chicken, another honey something. Under the sauce, the same battered chunks and the same fryer fat show up again and again. The names change. The parts do not.

This is the second kitchen at work, a hidden web of factories and freezers that powers much of what appears to be everyday life. You do not need to memorize every chemical name to see it. You only need to notice how your body feels after you eat from it.

> Here is what this chapter is asking you to do the next time you face a buffet or hot line:
> Remember, most choices are built from the same few factory parts wearing different costumes.
> Treat sauces and drinks as prominent players, not extras. They can drive symptoms as much as the fried food.
> Pay attention to what flares in your body after these plates, joints, stomach, sleep, or mood, and treat them as information, not bad luck.

You do not have to be perfect or swear off buffets forever. You can start by seeing past the shine and taking less from this second kitchen.

Once you learn to see through the buffet, it becomes much harder for the second kitchen to hide.

Chapter Three

Fryers, Oils, and Sauce Buckets

PULLING INTO THE DRIVE-THROUGH, warm salty haze used to signal comfort. Now my joints brace for impact. The sign outside promises variety and value. Behind the counter, steel pans glow under lamps, and fryers hiss in the background.

Years ago, this scene meant excitement: many choices, low prices, no dishes. After months of reading labels for "Poisoned at the Grocery Store," I cannot unsee what lives in the fryer and the sauce station. The crunch on a nugget or fry is not flour and heat.

It is a mix of cheap seed fat, factory-batch blends, preservatives, and flavor powders, built to last long shifts. Most fryers do not start each day with fresh oil. The same fat is heated, cooled, and reheated many times. Each cycle breaks it down a little more.

Damaged fats and off smells grow, and the kitchen covers them with more salt and seasoning. What started as a pale vegetable oil ends up as a dark bath that leaves everything with the same tired aftertaste. The food drops into the tub is just as engineered.

Coatings come from bags of dry mix; they read like lab notes rather than recipes. Starches, gums, leavening agents, colors, and flavor additives are blended so every batch fries the same. Chicken, fish, or a patty never met an animal that all get the same shell. By the time it hits your tray, you are eating the oil, the coating, and the chemistry, not just the potato or meat inside.

The sauce buckets stand ready to finish the job. Sweet and sour, barbecue, honey mustard, and special sauce are built from the same base: sugar or syrup, cheap oils, thickeners, salt, and artificial flavors and colors. Change the color and spice mix, swap a label, and yesterday's glaze becomes today's new item.

The menu might show flames, smoke, or fields of grain. The bucket in the cooler lists ingredients you would never keep in your own kitchen. Put the fryer and the sauce together, and you get the classic order. Something crispy plus something drenched.

It looks harmless a small side, a dipping cup, a quick treat. For a body already dealing with inflammation, blood sugar swings, or gout, this combo is closer to kindling and lighter fluid. The joint already hurts, the stomach already burns, the mind already feels dull; all have to cope with another round.

If your days include aching knees, stiff fingers, swollen feet, or a gut that never settles, you may not link your feelings to the fryers and sauce wells. You pass them without a thought. It is common to blame age, stress, or family history instead. The connection to daily food can be easy to overlook. Your body keeps sending a signal that something is off. Meanwhile, the usual order stays the same.

Crispy, salty, sweet, and dipped, everything is washed down with something sugary. The pills pile up, but the orders do not change.

Here is what this chapter wants you to see when you look at fryers and sauces:

The crunch is not cooking. It is often old, damaged oil that has been wrapped around a factory coating.

The dip is not a little extra. It can be a dense mix of sugar, cheap fats, and additives.

Your joints, gut, and energy may be reacting more to this fryer-and-sauce combo than to the plain food underneath.

You do not have to give up every fried bite forever. You can start by choosing it less often, skipping or reducing the number of sauces, and noticing how your body feels afterward.

In the next chapter, we move from what surrounds the food, the fat, and the sauce, to what lies inside the meat itself. You will see why the protein on the plate is not always the safest part of the meal.

Chapter Four

What Is Hiding in the Protein

EYES USUALLY GO STRAIGHT to the center of the plate when people judge a meal. Fries and dessert carry the guilt. A burger or grilled chicken feels responsible. Menus lean into instinct with the word 'protein' and phrases like 'premium' or 'flame-grilled'.

In reality, most animal products in everyday restaurants come from the same supply system that serves grocery stores. Hormones, drugs, feed, and processing tricks do not vanish when food enters a kitchen on the corner. Trust hide behind menu words instead of long labels.

For many chains and quick service spots, the animal's story starts in a feedlot or factory barn, not on pasture. Beef cattle are pushed to grow fast on genetically modified corn and soy sprayed with herbicides. Implants and drugs speed weight gain. Routine antibiotics help them survive in crowded pens.

Pigs and chickens live in large barns, and the blends help them grow and cope in tight spaces. By the time the result becomes a patty, nugget, strip, or slice, it carries the mark of a pharmaceutical farm more than of a field. After slaughter, more processing begins.

Trimmings, fat, and muscle are ground together and pressed into uniform shapes. Brines and injection pumps add water, salt, phosphates, and flavorings to keep the meat moist and springy during cooking. Poultry is minced and pressed into shapes that never existed on a living bird. Cheaper cuts get new names, such as steak tips or boneless wings.

Many products are treated with gases to hold color, tumbled in drums with sauces, then frozen and shipped. They are later reheated, grilled, or fried. The stripes on a sandwich may come from a real grill. They may also be printed marks on cooked portions that only need a quick warm-up.

Menu language helps cover the trail. A grilled chicken sandwich might start as breast pieces injected with broth, salt, and phosphates, then brushed with a sweet glaze and seared on a flat top. A signature burger could be ground from meat and fat from many animals, seasoned with flavor compounds, or washed with chemicals long before the restaurant sees it.

At many sit-down places, steak and pork arrive already soaked in bags of marinade. They sit in solutions designed to boost weight and tenderness, not nourishment. For human health, this layering matters.

Grain-fed feedlot beef tends to contain more pro-inflammatory fats than meat from animals raised on grass. It also has fewer protective fats and antioxidants. Heavy antibiotic use in these systems can promote the growth of resistant bacteria and may disrupt gut bacteria. Processed meats such as sausages, bacon, deli slices, hot dogs, and some burger blends often contain nitrites and other preservatives. Research links these additives to a higher cancer risk when they are eaten regularly.

Combine those proteins with fryer fat and sweet coatings from earlier chapters, and the protein becomes one more burden on joints, circulation, and liver rather than a shield. Portion size makes the load heavier. One sandwich may contain two or three standard servings of animal food.

Buffets invite multiple trips because diners feel they paid for the meat. Loaded appetizers, giant salads with bacon and poultry, and pasta piled with sausage and cream stack animal fat, processed tissue, white starch, and oils into a single hit. Over time, bodies respond with joint flares, chest tightness, morning stiffness, poor sleep, and a sense of being full but not nourished.

Not every restaurant serving is the same. Some independent places and a few chains do buy better meat from grass-fed cattle or pasture-raised birds, and they say so on the menu. When a dish names the farm and method, and the price matches effort, the picture improves. Without that kind of detail, the safest assumption is factory sourcing.

This book focuses on the baseline. The animal products most people eat most often do not come from special farms. They come from drive-through bags, cafeteria trays, and casual chain dinners, not from rare grass-fed steaks at a celebration.

When health care providers suggest cutting back on red meat or watching cholesterol, they are often reaching for a simple version of this story. What goes unsaid is how the animal's life, the processing steps, and the sauces and sides all shape the outcome.

A burger built from anonymous feedlot beef, cooked on shared equipment, topped with cheese and sweet sauce, hits the body in specific ways. Served with fried potatoes and a sugary drink, it strains blood sugar, digestion, and inflammation more than a simpler meal.

That mix does not behave like a simple, balanced meal once it is swallowed. It pushes blood sugar, strain, and inflammation much harder. It does not taste like a modest portion of slow-cooked meat with roasted vegetables at home.

Both plates may be called meat-based meals. On the surface, they can look similar. Inside the body, they create very different effects. The match in name hides a profound mismatch in impact.

On the surface, they can look similar. Inside the body, they create very different effects. They do not behave the same once swallowed. One meal pushes the body harder, while the other is gentler. Over time, those differences can add up.

Here is what this chapter wants you to remember when you look at the protein on your plate:

Do not assume the center is the healthy half just because it is labeled "protein".

If the menu does not tell you where the meat came from or how it was raised, it is from the factory system by default.

Processed meats, injected cuts, and heavily sauced or breaded proteins can contribute to inflammation and long-term health risks, especially when paired with fries and sweet drinks.

You do not need to quit meat entirely. Shifting toward smaller servings can change how your body responds. Choosing less processed options also helps. Home-cooked or clearly sourced dishes tell a different story.

In the following sections, we will see how these same patterns show up in institutional food and on children's trays. There, the second kitchen shapes bodies long before they ever walk into a buffet on their own. Those early patterns can echo through a lifetime.

Chapter Five

Feedlot in a Paper Bag

MOST PEOPLE PICTURE JUNK food as drive-through signs, crowns, buckets, mascots, and cars wrapped around a glowing window. Nobody mistakes it for health food. Yet for millions, it becomes breakfast, lunch, dinner, and snacks several times a week. As life speeds up, those paper wrappers start to feel less like an emergency stop and more like a food group.

Advertising tells a different story. Combo orders end in smiles and high fives, never in swollen fingers or a tight waistband. Burgers wear "100 percent beef" on the board. Poultry gets "all white meat." Fries promise "crisp and golden," and the word protein appears more than fat or sugar. Commercials show bright lettuce, red tomato, melted cheese, and steam rising from warm buns.

Nobody in those scenes looks tired, inflamed, or bloated afterward. Behind the picture, the same forces from earlier chapters show up again and again. Many sandwiches begin with animals raised in tight pens, pushed to gain weight on modified grains, growth drugs, and constant medication, rather than on pasture and time. The cow behind Patty lived in crowded yards, not on open grass.

Nugget pieces often started as birds packed into huge houses, breathing dust and growing so fast their legs strain under the load. By the time those parts reach the counter, the living creature has become a line on a purchase order. Patties hit flat tops slicked with cheap frying fat. Poultry drops into bubbling vats. Fish carries a coat of stripped flour and starch.

The fresh vegetables are thin slices laid over a stack built from vats, coatings, and bulk supply. The bundle leaves in a paper labeled "lunch." The body receives a dense mix of fat, fast starch, and extra compounds.

Portions expand along the way. A so-called small drink now looks like yesterday's medium, and free refills keep cups full with almost no thought. Fries get bumped up for a few cents. A sandwich can be made with extra patties, bacon, cheese, and special sauces. Bargain items stay cheap because real food would cost more.

Profit returns through volume, soda, and add-ons. Many people leave carrying more calories, sugar, and salt in one order than their grandparents did in a day. Trouble does not stop with the basket of fries.

Morning biscuit stacks can combine processed pork, cheese-like products, and bleached flour, followed by a flavored coffee drink with dessert-level sugar. Lighter wraps use white tortillas, factory fillings, and heavy dressings. Grilled choices often arrive coated in oil and sticky glaze: different menu names, the same heavy load for the body.

For anyone living with gout, high pressure, diabetes, or steady inflammation, these orders are far from neutral. They raise sugar, flood the system with sodium, and trigger inflammatory signals when the window stop happens several times a week. Joints complain, feet swell, sleep turns shallow, and energy crashes. The link to that glowing menu stays easy to ignore.

Blaming age, stress, or bad genes feels simpler than questioning the bag has become part of a daily routine. My own years in those lines followed the same arc. The window sat on the quickest route between inspections, and each order felt like another tool in my truck. Two fish sandwiches and fries, a burger, or a breakfast stack looked small next to crawl spaces, roofs, and paperwork.

Underneath, the beat was the same.—grease meat, sauces, white flour, sugar, repeat. My body tried to speak through my joints and my belly.

This does not mean every person must swear off drive-through food for life. It means phrases like "just a burger" or "just a quick lunch" hide what the bag really contains. Most orders combine factory-style animal products, fryer fat, stripped starches, and flavor boosters built for cravings, not for health. Once a kind of eating becomes weekly or daily, the damage stops hiding in the background and starts shaping a life.

Here is what this chapter wants you to see the next time you roll up to a glowing window:

That paper bag often holds feedlot meat, old fryer oil, white flour, and liquid sugar, not a quick bite.

The size of the drink, the extra patty, the sauces, and the value-add-ons can matter as much as the main sandwich.

If you live with pain, swelling, pressure issues, or sugar swings, these routine orders may be pushing your symptoms, not filling your schedule.

You do not have to quit fast food forever. Cutting visits can give your joints and vessels a different story to tell. Shrinking portions helps reduce the load as well.

Skipping some of the extras also eases the strain. In the pages ahead, the focus moves beyond the window lane to sit-down chains, buffets, cafeterias, and school food lines. It looks at the trays handed to children at school. Together, these places make up the rest of the second kitchen, which keeps calling this arrangement normal.

Chapter Six

Chain Restaurants in Fancy Clothing

MOST PEOPLE HEAR THE word "junk food" and picture drive-through signs and mascots. Sit-down chains with booths, servers, and dim lighting feel different. The menus are heavier, the plates are larger, and the prices are higher. The food can look closer to real cooking, with grill marks, herbs, and words like homestyle, artisan, or chef special.

Under a nicer outfit, much of the same second-kitchen machinery still runs. Many chain main dishes start with the same factory-raised animals, refined starches, and bulk sauces used in quick-service places. Boxes, bags, and pails arrive at the back door. They move into coolers and dry rooms, then onto plates in predictable steps.

The plate beneath the hanging lamp is often arranged in the same way as the items you have seen in paper bags. A homestyle chicken dish might be made from pre-breaded cutlets, par-fried in a plant, frozen, then finished in the restaurant fryer or oven. A glossy steak plate may rely on meat injected with brine to boost weight and tenderness, then brushed with a sweet glaze to create shine.

Pasta bowls that look generous and soothing can be mostly cheap noodles, processed cheese sauce, oil, and scattered bits of meat. The menu talks about comfort and tradition. The cartons talk about yield and holding time.

Portions often grow even more in these dining rooms. Starters arrive on platters meant to be shared, but one or two hungry people can easily eat them all. Main courses spill over the edges with meat, starch, and sauce. Refills on sweet tea, soda, or flavored lemonade keep sugar flowing quietly.

Value appears in larger plates, bottomless sides, and combo deals that stack heavy foods. For someone already dealing with joint pain, pressure issues, sugar swings, or steady inflammation, these outings are not neutral social events. A typical chain meal might include bread or chips to start, a loaded appetizer, a large meat-and-starch main dish, alcohol or sweet drinks, and dessert to share.

By the end of the night, the body has to handle a pile of factory meat, fryer fat, white starch, sugar, and alcohol in one sitting. The bill shows dollars. The body manifests as swelling, stiffness, and restless sleep.

The tricky part is that these places often feel like a step up from fast food. They are rewards after hard weeks, family traditions, and places to celebrate or connect. That emotional layer makes it harder to question what is actually on the plate. Saying no to a drive-through can feel practical. Saying no to a birthday dinner can feel disloyal, even if your knees and toes are already protesting.

This chapter is not asking you to avoid every family dinner or office gathering. It is asking you to see chain meals for what they are. One more major pipe feeding the second kitchen into your life, dressed in warmer light and nicer words.

Here are a few things to remember the next time you sit under a hanging lamp and open a thick menu:

Bigger plates and fancy language do not change where the items come from. Many are still factory-sourced and heavily processed.

Starters, sides, and drinks can add as much strain as the main dish, especially when they are fried, creamy, or loaded with sugar.

If you live with pain, swelling, or metabolic problems, these special nights can quietly become regular hits your body must absorb.

You do not have to stop going. Choosing simpler plates, skipping some extras, sharing portions, and limiting sweet drinks can turn these meals into actual celebrations rather than setbacks.

When you can see the second kitchen even in the nicest looking spots, it becomes easier to protect your body without giving up every social meal.

Chapter Seven

Kids, Cafeterias, and Vending Machines

FOR MANY CHILDREN, THE second kitchen does not start at a drive-through window. It starts in the lunch line. Trays slide along a rail past pans of nuggets, pizza squares, hot dogs, tater tots, and bright drinks. Posters on the wall show smiling kids, cartoon fruit, and slogans about strong bodies and sharp minds.

Nobody in those pictures looks tired, wired, or sick to their stomach after lunch. From a distance, the choices can look balanced. There is usually some protein, a starch, a vegetable, a fruit, and milk or juice. Look closer at what actually lands on a tray.

The protein might be breaded chicken made from minced meat and skin, pressed into shapes, and partly fried in a plant. The vegetable may be fried. The fruit could be canned slices in heavy syrup. Milk is often flavored and sweetened. Machines nearby fill gaps with chips, cookies, sports drinks, and energy beverages in bright wrappers.

Behind the sneeze guards and smiley posters, the same second kitchen system is doing its work. Frozen boxes of nuggets, patties, and pizza arrive from factories. Sauces come in pails and packets. Breads and buns are made from stripped flour and shortening.

Many schools and workplace cafeterias run on tight budgets. They lean on the cheapest, most stable items they can buy in bulk. The result is a steady flow of ultra-processed food into both small and grown bodies.

For children, this effect can be powerful. The school day is long. Many kids arrive hungry from rushed mornings or thin pantry options at home. If breakfast is sugary cereal, a sweet drink, and a muffin, and lunch is a breaded main with fries and chocolate milk, sugar swings hard before the final bell.

Some kids get labeled as unfocused, moody, or with behavioral problems when their bodies are simply reacting to what they were fed. Adults in cafeterias are not spared. Hospital staff, factory crews, office workers, and students move through similar lines.

They choose from steam-table favorites that look familiar and soothing. Pasta with cream sauce, breaded cutlets, loaded baked potatoes, pizza, burgers, and grab-and-go sandwiches all lean on the same oils, refined starches, processed meats, and sauces described earlier. Machines fill the gaps between shifts with candy bars, pastries, and energy drinks that hit fast and fade quickly.

Over time, this setting trains taste and expectation. Children learn lunch comes from a line, on a tray, with something breaded and something sweet. Workers get used to eating whatever fits into a short break and a tight budget. Packing food from home can feel strange, heavy, or even embarrassing compared to everyday cafeteria meals.

Meanwhile, knees, bellies, and minds keep a separate record. Heartburn after pizza day, afternoon crashes after syrupy drinks, and headaches after a lunch from a machine. This chapter is not about blaming schools, hospitals, or parents trying to stretch dollars and minutes.

It is about seeing cafeterias and machines as major branches of the second kitchen, feeding people who often have little control over the menu. When you see small changes become easier to defend.

Here are a few ideas to keep in mind the next time you or a child faces a tray line or a wall of machines:

Trays and snacks that look normal may still be built from the same factory meats, oils, and stripped starches as fast food.

For kids and shift workers, these plates are not rare treats. They can be a daily fuel, significantly affecting energy, focus, and long-term health.

Even in tight settings, small swaps can make a real difference. Choosing plain milk instead of flavored milk can help. Reaching for water instead of soda also matters. Picking fewer breaded items lowers the load. Bringing a straightforward item from home can change how a day feels.

Seeing school and workplace food as part of the second kitchen, not separate from it, makes it easier to question it. It also becomes easier to work around it. When possible, you can push for better options. When you understand how early and how often the second kitchen reaches into cafeterias and machines, typical kid and adult food starts to look very different. The choices that are still within reach begin to look different, too.

Chapter Eight

When Normal Food Makes You Sick

By now, the pattern should look familiar. Fast food, chain spots, buffets, cafeterias, and vending areas all draw from the same pantry. Factory meats, stripped starches, seed fats, sugar, salt, and additives repeat under different logos. Your knees, gut, heart, and brain do not care which sign hangs outside. They only respond to what reaches the blood.

Researchers call much of this ultra-processed food. These are products made primarily from extracts and factory-made ingredients, with very little whole food left. Frozen nuggets, fries, boxed pizzas, sweet cereals, chips, candy bars, many sauces, and diet drinks all belong to this group. So do many burgers, breakfast sandwiches, and school items. Extensive studies show the same pattern. The more ultra-processed food people eat, the higher their risks of weight gain, type 2 diabetes, high blood pressure, abnormal blood fats, and heart trouble.

One review found that people who eat the most ultra-processed items face much higher risks of diabetes, high blood pressure, unhealthy cholesterol patterns, and obesity. Those who eat the least of these foods face a lower risk.

Each additional serving was linked to worsening health markers, such as blood pressure and weight gain. Over time, those changes can build into serious problems. Together, these findings suggest that cutting back, even a little, can matter.

Each additional serving was linked with more pressure spikes and heart events. It was also tied to higher chances of cancer, gut disease, and death from any cause. These foods pack in energy but lack vitamins, minerals, and protective plant compounds. They push up weight and metabolic stress while real nourishment lags.

Ultra-processed food also stokes inflammation. It rapidly spikes blood sugar and triggers repeated insulin surges. It often delivers ample doses of omega-6-rich oils, salt, and additives that irritate the gut and blood vessels. Over time, a low but steady inflammatory state has been linked with heart disease, some cancers, fatty liver, kidney damage, and autoimmune problems. It rarely feels like one big event. It feels like waking up stiff, adding pills, and hearing your numbers are a little worse each year.

The effects do not stop at the waistline or the artery wall. Several studies have found that people who eat more ultra-processed food report more depression and anxiety. They also face higher risks of developing depression over time. Likely drivers include unstable blood sugar, inflammation, and shifts in gut bacteria. Diets built on these products often lack vegetables, fruit, nuts, and fish, which support brain health. When plates mostly come from boxes and bags instead of cutting boards and pans, the mood often follows the same roller coaster as blood sugar.

You do not need to memorize all these numbers to know something is wrong. You can feel it in your own body. If your joints flare, your stomach swells, your sleep gets worse, or your mood sinks after certain dishes, that is data. If those problems became more common as you ate out more and cooked less, it is a pattern. Labels and studies give names and percentages to what your body has been saying in plain pain for years.

For people like me with gout and diabetes, the pattern is even sharper. Fried foods, sweet drinks, processed meats, and white-flour plates are known triggers for flares and spikes in blood sugar. When those foods come from restaurants and buffets, they often arrive in larger servings and more concentrated forms than at home. A night out can mean a three-day limp. A treat dinner can mean morning sugar readings that belong on a warning label.

Add chronic inflammation, and every joint and organ has more work to do. This chapter is not here to scare you with statistics. It is here to connect the plates we have been talking about with the aches, labels, and bottles that follow. The second kitchen does more than fill your stomach.

Food shapes your weight, blood sugar, blood pressure, fat levels, mood, and pain over the years. Turned up, it can turn getting older into a slow slide toward stiffness and fog. Even when turned down, the same influence can make aging feel more like a steady walk than a fall.

For now, it is enough to accept this: your body is not betraying you. It is responding to what it has been fed. If your life has been built on restaurant dinners, buffets, cafeterias, and machines, your symptoms make sense. The good news is that changing the inputs can start to change the story.

Chapter Nine

Food, Fog, and Soul

For a long time, I treated pain as a glitch, not a message. If my toe hurt, I thought the toe was the problem. If my knees ached, I blamed the stairs. If I felt drained or moody, I blamed work, traffic, or other people. Food sat in a separate box. It was just something I grabbed to keep going.

Years of limping, stomach trouble, sugar swings, and brain fog finally got my attention. What sat on my plate was not shifting lab numbers. It was changing how I felt through every hour of the day.

After heavy restaurant meals, fast food, or buffets, I started to see a pattern. I was slower to think and quicker to snap. I had less patience with my kids. I did not feel like writing or fixing things around the house. My world shrank to the next task, the next couch, the next screen.

The gout and swelling were obvious. Underneath them was a dullness that felt like someone had turned down my inner dimmer switch. Once I saw it, it was hard to unsee.

Science does not use words like soul, but it does describe states most people would call fog and heaviness. Diets high in stripped starch, sugar, and damaged fats are linked with unstable blood sugar, ongoing inflammation, and poor sleep. Those three, in turn, are tied to more fatigue, more pain, and higher risks of depression and anxiety. When sugar keeps spiking and crashing, and your body is quietly on fire inside, it is hard to feel calm, present, or grateful. You are busy trying to drag yourself through the day.

It is not only the chemicals or the energy that count. It is also the constant distraction they create inside your own skin. A swollen or churning stomach pulls attention inward. Throbbing joints steal focus. A mind that feels packed with cotton makes simple tasks harder than they should be.

In that state, people reach for quick comfort. Another takeout order, another stop at a drive-through, another drink, another sweet snack. The second kitchen feeds the pain, and the pain feeds the second kitchen. Awareness gets pushed aside.

Sending most meals out to restaurants, chains, cafeterias, and machines also raises awareness. Someone else decides what is available, how it is cooked, and what is added. Your job is to pick from a list and pay. Food fades into background noise, something that happens while you work, drive, watch, and scroll.

It stops being a conscious ritual. It becomes a service you buy. The more you live that way, the easier it is to forget every bite is chemistry and energy for your cells and your thoughts.

In many older cultures, meals were treated as sacred time. People gathered, cooked, and ate with intention, prayers, and thanks. They knew where the food came from, who grew it, and what it took to bring it home. Today, many people eat alone in cars, at desks, or in front of screens, chewing on products whose origins they do not know.

The loss is not only nutritional. It is a loss of connection, of rhythm, and of the small daily moments when body and mind are in the same place. None of this means you must chant over every carrot or move into a monastery kitchen. It means that food is one of the most direct ways you meet the world, every day, whether you notice or not.

When most meals come from the second kitchen built on ultra-processed inputs, they shape more than weight and joint comfort. Mood, attention, and the basic sense of living comfortably inside your own skin all get pulled along. That slide becomes a spiritual concern as much as a medical one.

For me, the turning point came when I started treating food pain and fog as messages instead of random curses. When I noticed I could think more clearly and feel less inflamed after simple home-cooked meals, it felt as if someone had opened a window. I began to see each choice as a small vote for more clarity or more fog, more presence or more numbness.

It did not happen overnight, and I still make mistakes, but the frame shifted. Food stopped being only good or bad. It became part of learning to listen to my own body.

If you see yourself in these pages, you can take the same step. You do not have to become perfect or pure. You can start by noticing how you feel after restaurant meals, buffets, or heavy takeout, and comparing it to how you feel after simpler food at home. You can start by reclaiming one meal a day by preparing it with awareness rather than just ordering.

Each time you do that, you are doing more than changing calories. You are practicing attention. You are telling your body and your soul, "I am listening now."

In the chapters that follow, we will look at ways to do this without turning food into another source of stress. For now, it is enough to see that what you eat out there is not only building or breaking your health. It is also shaping how awake you can be to your own life.

Chapter Ten

One Meal Back in Your Hands

At this point, you might feel two things at once. One voice says, "This explains so much. This is my life." Another says, "Now what? I cannot quit restaurants, buffets, cafeterias, and machines tomorrow." That second voice is right. This is not a book about flipping your life overnight.

It is about an initiation. You wake up to what food has been doing to you, and you take back your choices, one small step at a time. If your days are anything like mine, restaurant food and takeout are woven into your routine. Work, kids, bills, traffic, fatigue, and tight money do not vanish because you read about oils and factory meat.

You still have early mornings, late nights, and people to feed. The idea of cooking three perfect plates a day for the rest of your life is enough to make anyone lie down with a pizza. So this chapter is not about perfection. It is about reclaiming enough ground that your body and soul can start to feel the difference.

A simple place to begin is with one meal. Not all of them. One. Pick the meal that feels most realistic for you to change. For many people, breakfast is the only time, because evenings are full and messy. For others, it is dinner, because mornings are a blur, but nights have a little more space.

Whichever you choose, let meal be yours again. Not the second kitchen's. Yours.

That meal need not be fancy. Simple is better. Eggs with some vegetables and fruit. Oatmeal with nuts and berries instead of sweet cereal. A bowl of soup and a salad. A baked potato with beans and a side of frozen vegetables.

A piece of real meat or fish cooked in your pan, with rice and something green. The goal is not gourmet. It is "I can clearly see what this is and mostly say the ingredients." Each time you eat a particular kind of food, notice how you feel that day and the next morning.

Eating out will still happen. Perfection is not the goal. In those moments, small shifts can ease the load on your body without turning you into the difficult person at the table. One simple move is to avoid fried foods plus heavy sauces in the same dish. Choose either fried or drenched, not both.

You can choose water instead of a sweet drink, or cut sugar by choosing unsweetened tea or diluting juice. You can order smaller portions, share main dishes, or take half home instead of clearing every large plate. You can look for plates built around a piece of real meat or fish, with fewer coatings and fewer mystery sauces.

These changes will not turn a chain restaurant into a monastery kitchen. They will begin to reduce the impact of damaged fats, sugar, and ultra-processed coatings that drive inflammation, sugar swings, and fog. If you have gout, diabetes, high pressure, or chronic pain, even these small moves can mean fewer flares and somewhat better mornings. That is not a theory. It is what many bodies report when people experiment.

One of the most powerful tools you can use now involves no exceptional food at all. It is paying attention and writing things down, not in a harsh, punishing way, but as listening. You can keep a tiny notebook or a note on your phone with two short lines each day. "What I ate was mostly real food." "How I felt the next morning."

Over a few weeks, patterns will start to appear. Certain places may always leave you limping. Some buffets might reliably bring a rough night of sleep. A week with more home cooking may give you steadier energy. That information belongs to you. No expert can feel it for you.

Think of this as a spiritual practice disguised as a practical one. You are training yourself to stay awake to your own life in the most physical way possible. Each time you cook something simple instead of ordering something complicated, you are practicing saying no to comfort and yes to awareness heals.

Each time you notice how your body responds, instead of numbing out or blaming age, you treat your pain as a teacher instead of an enemy. You will still have days when you grab fast food or eat from a buffet. Life will still throw you window emergencies, school meetings, and long workdays in strange places.

The point is not to scrub your record clean. It is to shift the balance slowly so more of your plates are ones you choose with your eyes open and your hands involved. Over time, those small shifts can change how your joints feel, how clearly you think, how you sleep, and how you show up with the people you love.

In the chapters ahead, we will look at how these small moves add up over months and years. The aim is to build a life where the second kitchen becomes an occasional tool, not the main fuel line. For now, remember this: you do not have to fix your whole story today. Taking one meal back into your own hands and noticing what changes is enough to begin.

Chapter Eleven

When Small Changes Start to Talk Back

AT FIRST, CHANGING ONE meal feels too small to matter. The restaurants are still there. The drive-through signs still glow. The school cafeteria and machines still surround you and your family. It is easy to think, "What difference can one home-cooked breakfast or one simple dinner make against all of that?" The answer shows up only if you stay with it long enough for your body to talk back.

For many people, the first signs are quiet. Maybe the toe throbs after certain dishes, but stays calmer one morning. Perhaps the scale moves a pound or two without a fight. Maybe you notice you are not as desperate for coffee in the afternoon when lunch was clean and straightforward. The changes are not fireworks. They are more like someone nudging the dimmer switch a little higher on your inner lights.

You do not get a new body in a week. You get small pieces of your old self back.

As weeks go by, patterns sharpen. You might notice that the pain and stiffness don't feel as constant when you have several days in a row with fewer fried, heavy restaurant plates. Sugar numbers may start to drift downward, or at least swing less wildly. Pressure might ease a bit. Clothes might feel looser.

None of this turns you into a magazine cover. It means your chemistry is not being pushed in the wrong direction as hard every day. Your joints, vessels, liver, and brain get a little more space to breathe.

Mood and clarity often shift, too. On days with more real food and fewer ultra-processed hits, thoughts may feel less foggy. You might snap less at minor annoyances and find a bit more patience with your family. Sleep can also improve when late-night restaurant food becomes less common. Waking up may feel more like climbing out of a shallow pool than clawing out of glue.

Choose one meal this week to cook or prepare yourself.

These are not miracles. They are the natural result of a body that is no longer being repeatedly hammered by the same mix of sugar, damaged fats, and additives.

Right now, set a reminder on your phone titled "My one meal" for tomorrow. For the next 14 days, give that reminder one small answer.

Each morning, rate your stiffness, pain, or fog from 0 to 5 on any scrap of paper or a phone note. Jot what you ate for that one meal beside it.

It is important to say clearly that you will still have setbacks. There will be weeks when work explodes, money gets tight, or life knocks you sideways, and the second kitchen rushes back in as the most straightforward answer. You may find yourself back at the buffet, in the window lane, or ordering three nights in a row before you realize what happened.

That does not erase your progress. It reminds you that the old patterns are still close at hand. The more profound shift is that you now notice how those weeks feel, and you know how to start turning the ship again.

Over time, what changes most is not only your numbers or symptoms, but your sense of who is in charge. Instead of feeling like a passenger fed by whatever the world offers, you begin to feel like someone who can choose, even if only part of the time. You learn which plates make you limp and which ones leave you steady. You know which meals fog your mind and which ones clear it.

That knowledge is not abstract. It is written in your knees, your sleep, and your mornings.

For some people, this becomes the start of a new identity. You are no longer just "someone with bad genes" or "someone who loves junk food." You become someone who listens to their own body and decides accordingly. Not perfectly. Not without struggle.

That kind of honesty is part of the initiation this book has been pointing toward. It marks the moment you stop waiting for a pill, a plan, or a miracle to rescue you. Instead, you begin working with the information your own life has been offering all along.

The outside world may not be built for ease. The second kitchen will still call your name. For now, taking one meal back into your own hands is enough. If you notice even small shifts in pain, energy, or mood, that single change already matters. It is your body saying, "I see this. I like this. Keep going."

Fast Rules for One Better Meal

For your one meal, eat from a real plate, not a bag or box.

Make half the plate something that once looked like a plant, not a powder.

Stop when you feel gently full, even if there is food left.

Chapter Twelve

Poisoned at the Drive Through: Why the Restaurant Will Not Save You

Most people do not walk into a restaurant thinking, "I am here for a dose of pesticides, seed fats, and mystery meat." They walk in hungry, tired, and hopeful. The light is warm, the menu is friendly, and plates that pass by look like small works of art. The mind relaxes. "Someone else is cooking. I am safe here."

The hard truth is that, in most places, the real difference between a store and a restaurant is location. Boxes open in the back, the chemicals are heated, and you receive them on a plate rather than from your own refrigerator. There is no secret garden behind most dining rooms, only a loading dock and a dumpster.

Most places are not pulling carrots from the oil or walking to a pond to catch fish. They order from the same large distributors that supply grocery chains, hospitals, nursing homes, and stadiums. Trucks back up to the door carrying pallets of frozen meat and fish, boxes of precut vegetables, tubs of sauces, and cases of desserts.

Many items have already traveled long distances from industrial farms, feedlots, and fish pens that you will never see. A local favorite might buy napkins or decor nearby. The food itself often follows the same price path as the market's cheapest item.

A simple plate that sounds harmless, grilled chicken, salad, bread, and a side, can carry more chemistry than you would guess. The chicken may come from a large confinement barn, raised on modified grain and given regular medications. It may then be injected or tumbled in brines and phosphates to keep it moist and heavy. What looks simple on the plate can be pretty complex behind the scenes.

The salad greens likely come from large fields treated with weed killers, insecticides, and fungicides, then washed, bagged, and shipped through refrigerated warehouses. The bread is made from refined flour, sugar, industrial fats, conditioners, and preservatives, not flour, water, yeast, and salt.

The dressing, which looks like olive oil and herbs, often starts life in a large bucket. It is thickened with gums and emulsifiers, then sweetened, colored, and preserved. All of this helps it still look perfect after weeks in a cooler.

Restaurants, ghost kitchens, and institutional kitchens all live on these bulk goods. Behind the swinging doors are not just baskets of freshly picked tomatoes. There are boxes labeled with technical names such as sodium tripolyphosphate, carrageenan, xanthan gum, modified starch, natural flavors, colorants, and preservatives. These are the same types of ingredients you saw in the grocery store book.

What looks like a simple meal is made up of many industrial components. Each part has been designed to last, travel well, and remain eye-catching and appealing. The result is that food feels familiar but is far from home cooking. Over time, those hidden additions can change how the body feels.

Fast Rules When You Eat Out

Start with water, not soda, while you read the menu.

Skip combos that stack fries, bread, and dessert on the same order.

Ask for sauce or dressing on the side once each day you eat out.

Home-style gravy may come from a bag. Signature sauces often begin as processed bases trucked in from afar. The sign may say "made from scratch," but unless your kitchen uses stabilizers and giant buckets, "scratch" is being defined loosely.

Even with better ingredients, the cooking fat can still cause trouble. Many kitchens rely on large vats of cheap seed oils such as soybean, canola, corn, or cottonseed. These stay in heavy rotation on flat tops and in fryers because they cost less and can be used all day. They are heated and reheated, breaking down into oxidized fats and reactive compounds that irritate blood vessels, stress the liver, and drive ongoing inflammation.

Fries, wings, fish, onions, and even vegetable sides share the same tired oil. The grill marks on a piece of fish might be real. The history of the thin oil film on the flat top is not something anyone prints on the menu.

All of this would be bad enough if it were only about energy or too much fat. It is not. For a body already dealing with gout, arthritis, diabetes, high pressure, or brain fog, each restaurant plate can act like a small chemical and inflammatory event. Industrial oils and oxidized fats can raise inflammation, leading to more swelling, more morning stiffness, and more pain in sensitive joints. Processed meats and poultry, loaded with phosphates, nitrites, and salt, put extra strain on the kidneys, blood vessels, and heart.

The burden grows when they keep showing up in breakfast stacks, deli piles, pizzas, and loaded starters again and again. The gut takes a beating, too. Emulsifiers and thickeners, such as carrageenan, polysorbates, carboxymethylcellulose, xanthan, and guar gum, help keep sauces and dressings creamy and stable during storage.

Regular exposure to some emulsifiers has been linked to disturbed gut microbes, a thinner mucus layer, and low-grade inflammation in the gut wall. When the barrier is irritated, people often notice more bloating, unpredictable bathroom trips, fatigue, and a foggy head after plates that were supposed to be light or healthy. The brain does not float above this. It sits at the end of the same bloodstream, getting whatever the gut and liver cannot handle.

Sugar and pressure also pay a price. Restaurant food often stacks refined starches, hidden sugar, and large portions in a single meal. That mix enters the bloodstream quickly and triggers a surge of insulin. Over time, the rise-and-crash pattern contributes to insulin resistance, weight gain around the middle, and the tired-but-wired feeling never quite goes away. Salt is poured freely, not because cooks are villains, but because sugar and salt are cheap ways to make almost anything taste better and keep people coming back.

For someone whose pressure is already creeping up, a steady habit of salty, additive-heavy plates becomes fuel for the same problems pills are trying to control. Then there is the slow, quiet chemical load nobody orders but everybody gets. Pesticide residues on produce, contaminants in farmed fish and factory-farmed meat, preservatives in processed cuts, and compounds from packaging all end up on restaurant plates.

Metal cans, plastic liners, coated cardboard, and grease-resistant paper can leach substances into sauces, soups, and fried foods when heated and when fat is present. No one has tested exactly what happens when a human body eats mixtures of these compounds three times a day for decades. We do know long-term higher exposure to some pesticides, preservatives, and pollutants is linked with higher risks of cancer, metabolic disease, and gut disorders.

For years, it has been easy to tell yourself you are doing better by eating out instead of buying junk food. The bill feels more grown-up than a frozen pizza, and the plate looks more respectable. That was my story too. It felt like an upgrade to avoid the grocery aisles and sit at a table with a menu.

In reality, all that changed was who opened the boxes. The same factories, farms, and chemical suppliers fed the kitchen. The same seed fats and additives ran the show. I was spending more money to be poisoned at the company than I would have been alone.

This is not a call to swear off every dining room for life. It is a call to drop the illusion that a tablecloth or a clever menu name makes food safe. A plate can be beautiful and still be made from sprayed vegetables, factory-raised animals, farmed fish, reheated industrial fats, and a long list of hidden additives. The restaurant will not save you, because it eats from the same trough as the grocery store, then hides the evidence under sauce and lighting.

The scary part is not only what happens in the kitchen. It is what happened before the truck ever backed up to the door. The chickens did not start their lives under heat lamps near a strip mall. The fish did not hatch in the freezer truck. The bright vegetables did not grow under the glow of the salad bar.

They began on farms, in feedlots, in fish pens, and in fields sprayed and dusted with chemicals, but never made it onto the menu. If restaurant food is the performance, farming is the rehearsal. The real story of pesticides, metals, and engineered crops starts there, in places most diners never see and never think to ask about.

In the next chapter, we will move back upstream, past plates and buffets, to the places where food begins. We will return to soil, spray rigs, fish farms, and feed bins to see what really rides along on every healthy-looking bite.

Chapter Thirteen

Beautiful Food, Sick Body: Poisons from Field to Plate

You can stand in front of a buffet and see nothing but beauty. Shiny trays. Bright colors. Greens look crisp, meats that glisten, fruit could be on a card. Your eyes whisper, "This has to be good for me. Look at it." That is the trick. In this system, food is designed to look safe and abundant while carrying hidden harm.

The poison does not announce itself with a skull and crossbones. It rides in on bright lettuce, polished apples, thick steaks, pink fish, perfect bread, and golden fries. The problem starts long before the restaurant or market. It begins in the field and the feedlot, in the fish pen and the spray rig.

Most food that ends up on a plate in front of you comes from industrial farms and factories whose first job is not health. It is volume, price, and appearance. Crops are bred and engineered to survive shipping and look good on shelves, not to be rich in minerals or flavor. Fields are sprayed with weed killers, bug killers, and mold sprays.

The plant survives. The pests die. The chemicals do not vanish. Tiny leftovers cling to the skin and sink into the flesh. Wash water and pretty displays do not change the story written in soil.

Animals are treated the same way. Cattle, pigs, and chickens are raised in crowded barns and feedlots, where the main concerns are feed efficiency, growth rate, and disease prevention. Their feed is often made from modified grains grown with the same sprays used on corn and soy fields. When sickness threatens, drugs step in.

During processing, more layers are added. Solutions, phosphates, nitrites, flavor enhancers, and tenderizers keep everything moist, pink, and tasty on the plate. By the time the steak, chicken breast, or burger reaches you, it is not an animal product. It is an animal plus everything the system poured into it along the way.

Fish wears an even stronger halo. Fresh catch. Light and healthy. Heart smart. But much of the fish on modern plates never saw wild rivers or open oceans. It grew in crowded pens or tanks, fed pellets made from other industrial ingredients, and swam in water collected waste, chemicals, and sometimes plastic bits.

Wild fish, when they do appear, have spent years filtering whatever their waters now carry. Metals, runoff, and other pollutants do not make the fish look sick. They make the fish look normal while the people who eat them grow sick.

Grain and flour tell the same story in another form. Wheat, corn, and rice are grown on depleted soils, pushed to yield with synthetic fertilizers and weed killers. Once harvested, they are stripped, ground, bleached, and milled into flours that perform well in machines but poorly in human bodies. Vitamins and minerals are added back in lab forms to make the label look reassuring.

Then those flours become bread, pasta, cakes, pastries, batter, coatings, cereals, and snacks. On the outside, it looks like comfort: a warm roll, a soft bun, a beautiful slice of cake. On the inside, you are eating starch that slams your sugar like a fire, plus residues and additives from each step of its journey.

The cruel part is how ordinary it all feels. You can sit at a table with friends and look at your plate with pride. "I ordered the salad. I chose fish instead of a burger. I picked the whole-grain bread." You did your best with the story you were told.

Meanwhile, the lettuce may have been grown on a field that sees more chemicals in one season than your grandparents saw in a decade. The fish may carry a quiet cargo of pollutants and farm compounds. The whole-grain bread may contain refined flour, sugar, coloring, and seed fat. The food looks honest. The supply chain behind it is not.

For someone already dealing with gout, arthritis, diabetes, high pressure, or constant fatigue, this matters. Your joints do not care how pretty the plate is. Your vessels do not care how good the menu sounds. Your gut and liver only see what arrives. Sprays that irritate and confuse, metals and pollutants that burden clearance, stripped starches that hammer sugar, and oils that feed the fire of inflammation.

You can follow every slogan. "Eat more fish." "Eat more salads." "Choose whole grains." You can still feel worse. The food living under those labels has been changed.

This is why so many people feel like they are doing everything right and still getting sicker. They buy beautiful fruit that traveled far and has been sprayed many times. They order grilled fish that has been grown up in a chemical bath. They pick bread that promises fiber and heart health but is made with factory flour and sugar. The illness that follows is blamed on age, genes, or bad luck, while the daily stream of altered food goes unchallenged.

The system has become skilled at making unhealthy food look like the answer to health. There is a reason your body sometimes reacts as if it has been ambushed after a week of good choices. The toe throbs again. Knees swell. Pressure creeps up. Sleep worsens. Fog thickens.

You may tell yourself, "I have been so careful. I have eaten so well." The truth is more complex. You have eaten what the system calls 'healthy,' but it has been poisoning its own definition of 'healthy' for decades.

The point of this chapter is not to say every apple is dangerous or every farm is corrupt. It is to open your eyes to the gap between how food looks and what it contains. Until you see that gap, it is easy to blame yourself, your willpower, or your genes for illness that has been built into the supply chain.

Once you see it, you can stop being shocked that beautiful food has made you sick. You can start asking better questions. Where did this come from? What was it fed? What was sprayed on it? How far did it travel? Who handled it? Most of all, how much of my plate can I bring back into my own hands?

In the chapters ahead, we will look more closely at these hidden layers, including plant sprays, metals in soil and water, and engineered crops that keep the machine running. The goal is not to turn you into a chemist. It is not to make you into a farmer either. Instead, the aim is to give you enough clear sight for daily choices. That way, when you look at a plate of great-looking food, you can also hear what your knees, gut, liver, and mind have been trying to say for years.

Chapter Fourteen

Poisoned at Home: The Second Kitchen in Your House

At home, the second kitchen does not knock. It slips in through boxes, cans, bags, and frozen bricks that promise fast, family-sized, and just heat-and-serve. You can stand in your kitchen at night and look around. Even when you are eating at home, a distant factory may still be doing most of the cooking.

The microwave clock glows, the freezer hums, and shelves sag under cardboard and plastic. This is not a crime scene kitchen from television. It is an ordinary house filled with ordinary food, slowly wearing down an ordinary body.

The second kitchen moves in for understandable reasons—pain, fatigue, time, and money. On days when joints hurt and sleep is poor, the box that says 'ready in 10 minutes' feels like mercy. When you stagger in from work, and your toe is screaming, the frozen pizza does not look like a villain. It seems like a lifeline.

When bills are tight, a case of canned soup, beans, or value dinners looks like a smart move. None of this means you are lazy or foolish. It means you live in a world where boxes and bags are built to slide into your life at its weakest points.

Open the pantry, and the second kitchen waves back in bright colors. Cereal boxes grin with mascots. Crackers talk about whole grains and heart health. Instant noodles promise comfort in minutes. Cake mixes, pancake mixes, boxed macaroni, flavored rice packets, stuffing, and helper kits line up.

Ingredient lists, when read, tell a different story. Stripped flours, several kinds of sugar, seed and palm fats, emulsifiers, gums, and flavorings. Colors, preservatives, and lab-made vitamins stand in for nutrients that should have come from soil. Some boxes and liners also carry grease-resistant coatings and other packaging compounds that can slowly move into the food, over time and with heat.

Canned food feels solid and honest. Metal, weight, a satisfying clunk on the counter. Soup, beans, chili, vegetables, fruit, pasta in sauce, canned meats. They sit for years in cupboards, waiting. Canning does preserve food, and simple canned items can be helpful.

But many modern cans hide linings made from industrial chemicals meant to resist rust and grease. Those coatings can contain hormone-disrupting compounds that are absorbed into whatever they come into contact with, acidic or fatty foods. Open a can of soup with an ingredient list as long as your arm, and you'll see more than vegetables and broth. The liquid inside is food plus whatever the lining has added along the way.

The freezer is the second kitchen's cold storage room. Open the door, and you may find pizzas, breakfast sandwiches, waffles, healthy frozen dinners, nuggets, fries, battered fish, burritos, and tubs of ice cream. Many of these products are built like restaurant plates, just frozen. Refined flours or starches, seed fats, processed meats, cheeses with anticaking agents, sauces thickened with gums and starches, preservatives, and colors to survive months in a box.

Cardboard and plastic wraps keep them neat and stackable. They can also carry grease-resistant coatings and other packaging compounds that can migrate into food over time and with heat—the box talks about garden vegetables and home-style cooking. The ingredient list and packaging tell you it has spent more of its life in warehouses and trucks than in any garden or home.

The refrigerator looks safer at first glance. Real jars. Real leftovers. Maybe real vegetables. Look closer, and the second kitchen sits on every shelf, takeout containers with cold fries and half-eaten sandwiches. Bottles of salad dressing are made from seed oils, sugar, salt, gums, and flavors. Coffee creamers are closer to flavored oil blends than dairy.

Delis meats and cheeses are preserved and stabilized with nitrites, phosphates, and anticaking agents. Healthy yogurts and drinks are sweetened and thickened so they feel rich and dessert-like. None of these things is evil in a single bite. The problem is that, for many people, breakfast, lunch, and dinner become the default, built from bottles, tubs, and trays rather than basic ingredients.

Living with a second kitchen inside your house has consequences. The same chemicals, additives, and industrial fats that caused trouble in restaurant plates keep showing up at home. Each time you stir powdered cheese into macaroni or heat boxed noodles, you feed your body refined starches, seed fats, colors, and preservatives that raise sugar and trigger inflammation.

Each can of thick, salty soup brings more than vegetables and meat. It also delivers compounds from the lining, refined starch, and a heavy dose of sodium. Each frozen pizza combines white flour, unstable fats, processed meats, and a long chain of additives in one convenient circle.

Over time, convenience can start to look like flares after easy dinners. Mornings with stiff, burning joints can follow a night of frozen comfort food. Sugar spikes can follow healthy frozen entrees. Poor sleep often trails a parade of take-and-bake specials.

A bit of dry humor can help you see this. Your pantry is not just a place to store food. It stores a small chemistry lab on every shelf. Some boxes have spent more time in a lab than your doctor. If a product has a mascot, a health claim, and a three-year shelf life, your joints should be nervous.

The words on the front tell stories about nature, family, and tradition. The small print on the back tells stories of factories, additives, and shelf-life engineering.

The goal is not to make you fear every can or box. Some canned beans, plain tomatoes, or frozen vegetables with simple labels can be helpful tools. The goal is to see which items belong to your kitchen and which belong to the second kitchen that has been living rent-free in your cupboards.

The good news is you do not have to evict the second kitchen overnight. You can start small. One shelf. One drawer. One meal. Swap a boxed side for potatoes or rice you cook yourself trade one frozen dinner for a pan of eggs and vegetables. Replace one bottle of thick sweet dressing with oil, vinegar, salt, and herbs.

Each time you do, you take a little ground back from the factories. You also give your joints, gut, liver, and brain a plate that looks more like food and less like a project from an industrial design team.

Your body has been trying to tell you about this second kitchen for a long time—the throbbing toe after a string of easy dinners. Fingers swell when frozen meals and canned soups become routine. The fog that follows nights of pizza and boxed snacks. None of it's random.

In the next chapter, the focus shifts to those signals themselves. Gout, joint pain, sugar swings, bathroom emergencies, fatigue, and fog. They form an early warning system your body has always had, long before any expert or label spelled it out.

Chapter Fifteen

The Healthy Meal That Was Not: What You Really Ordered

YOU SIT DOWN, DETERMINED to do better this time. No, all-you-can-eat buffet, no bottomless fries. Just a careful meal. You order a diet cola, a side salad with Thousand Island dressing and croutons, a quarter chicken, corn, a baked potato, and coffee with blueberry cheesecake.

This feels reasonable. It feels grown-up. It feels like something a doctor might accept. Then comes the question that this chapter is built on. What did you really order?

Start with the diet cola. It looks like the safe choice, no sugar, no energy, just bubbles, and taste. That taste is not coming from a mountain spring. It comes from acids, artificial sweeteners, color, and natural flavors mixed in a lab.

The caramel color in many colas is not caramel made in a home kitchen. It is an engineered color that has raised concern in some forms and doses when exposure is high and long. Artificial sweeteners such as aspartame, sucralose, or acesulfame potassium do not slip through the body like ghosts. Heavy, regular use can disturb gut bacteria and may alter how the body handles sugar, even when the label reads zero.

The acids bathe your teeth and can erode enamel over time. You ordered no sugar. You got a gut experiment and an acid wash.

Now look at the salad. Lettuce, a few vegetables, some croutons, Thousand Island dressing. It sounds almost virtuous. The lettuce and vegetables may already contain small amounts of sprays and residues from fields and washhouses.

The croutons are small chunks of industrial bread made from stripped flour, seed fats, sugar, conditioners, and preservatives, maybe with a dusting of cheese powder. The real act happens in the dressing. Thousand Island at most places is a mix of cheap seed oil, sweeteners, salt, vinegar, and a long list of gums, stabilizers, colors, and flavors.

The bottle or bucket it came from is designed for months of storage in a cooler, not for your arteries' health. You ordered something light on the side. You got a spray sampler with a sugar-and-oil chaser.

The quarter chicken arrives looking respectable. Skin browned, meat tender, maybe a shiny glaze. It is easy to imagine a farm somewhere in this story. The reality is more often a crowded barn and a processing plant.

The bird was likely raised in tight conditions on modified grains, with drugs in the feed to prevent disease from spreading. During processing, carcasses may be chilled in large communal baths where bacteria, chemicals, and water mix. To keep the meat moist and juicy, processors often inject or tumble solutions containing water, salt, phosphates, and flavorings.

Phosphates help retain water and improve texture, but they increase the load on your kidneys and vessels. If the skin is glossy and sweet, you also get sugar and more additives from a glaze or sauce. You ordered lean protein. You got an animal, plus everything the system fed, injected, and dipped it with.

Corn on the plate is a safe vegetable. It is familiar, bright, and tastes sweet. Most corn in the country comes from large fields where plants are engineered and treated with pesticides to control weeds and pests. The kernels do not reveal how many passes the sprayer made or what the runoff did downstream.

Corn is also a starchy side that breaks down into sugar, raising blood glucose levels. If it has been buttered with margarine or a vegetable oil spread instead of real butter, each bite also carries seed oils and emulsifiers. You ordered a vegetable. You got a sweet sprayed starch with oil on top.

The baked potato seems like the safest part of the plate. A whole potato, baked in its skin, feels honest. The potato itself, like the corn, grew in fields treated with fertilizer, weed killers, and mold sprays. The real trouble arrives with the toppings.

Butter is often replaced with margarine or blends made from seed fats, emulsifiers, flavors, and colors. Sour cream can be thickened with gums. Cheddar turns into cheese sauce built from processed cheese, fats, starch, and color. Bacon bits may be processed meat preserved with nitrites and smoked.

Load the potato, and you stack refined fats, processed meats, and additives on top of a large, fast-acting starch. You ordered a plain baked potato, maybe dressed up a little. You got a starch mountain dressed in seed fats, stabilizers, and factory meats.

After all that, dessert feels like surrender. "I already slipped, might as well enjoy this." Coffee and blueberry cheesecake arrive like old friends. The coffee itself can be simple if it is just beans and water, though the journey from bean to cup has its own story. The creamers and sweeteners bring another mix of seed fats, sugar or syrup, thickeners, and flavors.

The cheesecake is a beautiful triangle of everything this book has warned against. The crust is made from crushed cookies or crackers, which are refined flour, sugar, fats, and additives. The filling is cream cheese and sugar at best, but often includes stabilizers and whipped toppings made with industrial oils.

The blueberry topping is not just fruit. It is fruit plus sugar, syrup, colors, and flavors designed to stay bright and glossy. You ordered a small treat. You got a concentrated dose of sugar, refined starch, unstable fats, additives, and packaging-related compounds from how it was stored and shipped.

When the meal ends, you feel proud of skipping the fry parade and a little guilty about the cake. You ask for a container and take the leftovers home. The box or clamshell feels harmless, a thrifty move. Many of those containers are made of plastics, coated, or treated with grease-resistant agents that can leach compounds into hot, fatty food as it cools.

The warm package goes into your refrigerator, next to what you bought and cooked yourself. The second kitchen has just mailed more of its chemistry into your house, labeled as tomorrow's lunch.

Altogether, this careful meal looks nothing like a fast food binge. It is not a double burger with extra cheese and a bucket of fries. It is the kind of order people make when they are trying. That is what makes it such a strong example.

If this is what trying looks like in many restaurants, it is no surprise bodies stay inflamed. Sugar stays wild, guts stay upset, and minds remain foggy. The plate feels like it is doing better, but it is still built from industrial drinks, sprayed produce, factory meats, seed oils, stripped starches, and sugars. A long list of additives is still working in the background.

The point is not that you must never drink a diet cola or never look at cake again. The fact is, a menu can break your resolve with a few gentle words. The names on the page, salad, chicken, corn, baked potato, and blueberries, are costumes. Below, the same second kitchen and the same system are in operation.

Once you see what you really ordered at night, the spell starts to crack. You even carried some of it home in a plastic box for your own refrigerator. Afterward, it becomes harder to pretend that illness is merely bad luck or bad genes. It starts to look like the natural outcome of plates that were booby-trapped all along.

Chapter Sixteen

Your Body's Early Warning System

THIS IS THE CHAPTER where your body, in the end, gets to talk, and it does not whisper. Until now, the food has taken most of the attention. Menus, boxes, chemicals, and the second kitchen in your house have been center stage. Here, the spotlight turns around.

The throbbing toe, stiff knees, pounding head, bathroom emergencies, afternoon crashes, foggy thinking, and strange lab numbers have all been trying to speak. They use different languages but send the same basic message. Something you are eating is not working.

Careful reviews now show that eating more ultra-processed food raises the risk of heart disease, stroke, type 2 diabetes, weight gain, sleep problems, depression, and early death.

People who eat the most ultra-processed food can face much higher risks of dying from heart disease. They are also more likely to have several chronic conditions. That can mean cancer plus diabetes, or stroke plus heart disease.

The fun food and the healthy-looking processed food do more than tighten waistbands. They stack the deck toward sickness in several ways.

Zoom in closer, and the list of chemicals starts to sound like a supply catalog. Emulsifiers such as carboxymethylcellulose and polysorbate 80 are often used. They are found in sauces, dressings, ice cream, and baked goods. In lab and animal studies, they can thin the gut's mucus layer and alter the bacterial mix.

That mix of damage can trigger low-grade inflammation and move the body toward metabolic syndrome, obesity, and inflammatory bowel disease. Certain pesticides have been linked with higher risks of Parkinson's disease, Alzheimer's disease, and several cancers in exposed groups.

As bodies age, livers and kidneys clear these compounds more slowly. Residues that a younger person might handle can accumulate and cause greater harm in older adults. Add sweeteners, colors, preservatives, and oxidized oils, and each typical day starts to look like a slow chemistry experiment running inside your joints and organs.

Picture waking up after a week of being good. You skipped the obvious junk and ordered the salad with chicken. You chose the baked potato instead of fries and drank diet soda.

You reheated leftovers at home instead of heading back to the window. On paper, it looks better than before, but the morning does not match the script.

The foot throbs. Knees feel packed with sand. Fingers look puffier than last month. Your back aches, and crossing the room feels like walking on borrowed legs. Your head is thick, and bending to tie your shoes already sounds like work.

When this passes for a reward, the mind looks for a softer story. Maybe this is just age. Perhaps it is your genes. Perhaps this is how life feels now.

Doctors see you for ten or fifteen minutes. They note joint pain, high pressure, creeping A1C, odd cholesterol ratios, and say words like osteoarthritis, hypertension, prediabetes, metabolic syndrome, mild cognitive impairment, and irritable bowel. A pill for pressure, a pill for sugar, something for sleep, something for mood, plus advice to lose weight and avoid salt.

Very few ask how many emulsifiers, residues, artificial sweeteners, and reheated seed fats you ate this week. Even fewer connect a waddling walk, swollen fingers, and the need to lean on a cart for balance to a lifetime of ultra-processed food and restaurant chemistry. It is as if the whole system decided that what you eat is only about energy and salt, while the chemical storm riding on those calories passes unmentioned.

Look around any store or mall, and the results are out in the open. Older people shuffle, gripping carts or canes, faces set in a constant wince. Middle-aged people waddle more than walk, hips and knees turning like rusty hinges, shoulders slumped. Much of this gets blamed on wear and tear and old age, as if joints expire like batteries.

Joints sit at the crossing point of weight, inflammation, sugar, and the toxic load carried by cartilage, bone, and joint fluid. The more years a body spends bathing in oxidized seed fats, emulsifiers, pesticides, sweeteners, and ultra-processed flours, the louder those joints complain. Ever wonder why so many older people waddle rather than stride? A large part of the answer is decades of industrial food.

Their joints respond in the only way they can. They hurt.

Is this too much for one chapter? Not if the goal is to tell the truth. It does require honesty to take those labels seriously. Hypertension, type 2 diabetes, coronary artery disease, atrial fibrillation, fatty liver, gout, osteoarthritis, mild cognitive problems, depression, and irritable bowel are not random lightning strikes. Your food and its chemicals may have played a starring role.

This is not about blaming you for every illness. It is about refusing to pretend a lifetime of ultra-processed, dusted, and additive-loaded food has nothing to do with how hard it is to rise from a chair.

There is still space here for a little dry humor, because sometimes the only way to face this is with a crooked smile. Nobody told you that polysorbate eighty might help your gut leak like an old roof. No one mentioned certain sprays might have a cameo in your salad's past. Nobody stamped a big warning on emulsified heart-healthy dressings saying, "May promote metabolic problems if eaten daily."

Instead, we got happy cows on cereal boxes and berries on yogurt tubs, but met a real berry. Ads showed smiling people who somehow ate this way and still jogged at sunrise. So no, this is not too much for this section this is precisely where it belongs.

From here, the rest of this part can walk through each alarm on your body's control panel, including joint pain, gut trouble, brain fog, crashes, pressure, and sugar. It will show how meals loaded with these chemicals worsen each signal. The more of this food you eat, the less margin your body has left. As the years pass, your body can no longer absorb the hit. That is when everyday choices start to feel like heavy blows instead of harmless habits.

The liver and kidneys slow down—the gut lining thins. The microbiome grows more chaotic. The result is not just getting old, but becoming far more open to diseases that an honest food system would try to prevent, not quietly feed.

Chapter Seventeen

Blood Sugar on a Roller Coaster

IT WAS AN ATYPICAL morning on the way to an Amish produce auction. A bowl of cereal sat on the table, something you seldom ate, but one of the kids was having it, so you did too. About two hours later, walking around the auction, your feet started tingling and then turned to cotton. It felt as if the ground was there, but the signals from your nerves were wrapped in towels.

You sat down at the snack bar. The woman behind the counter took one look at you, pricked your finger, and said, "Sir, you are having a small diabetes reaction." She handed you a candy bar. The sugar pulled you out of the crash, and you felt your feet return.

One bowl, one strange episode, and a warning that something in your sugar wiring was already fragile. That same wiring takes another hit every time you eat a good-looking meal built from boxes, cans, bottles, squeeze bottles, and restaurant buckets.

The sugar roller coaster does not only show up after cereal. It seems that every time a plate is loaded with refined starches and sugar, they hit the bloodstream quickly. White breads and buns, croutons and breaded coatings, sweet dressings and sauces squeezed out of plastic bottles all feed the same spike. Ketchup, barbecue sauce, sweet chili sauce, desserts, light yogurts, and coffee drinks often taste like melted ice cream; they usually hide sugar to make them more addictive.

A typical restaurant-style day for many people looks like this. Breakfast on the go is a sweet coffee drink and a muffin or pastry. Lunch is a healthy sandwich or wrap on soft bread with a lovely drink. Dinner is a big plate with bread, pasta or potatoes, sauces, and dessert.

The result is a sugar pattern that looks like a jagged mountain range, up, down, up, down, all day. Each time one of these plates hits, sugar rises. The body floods the blood with insulin to pull sugar into cells.

For a while, there is a brief high, energy, comfort, a sense of being fed. Then, in bodies already strained by years of this pattern, sugar drops too far or too fast. That is when shakiness, irritability, sudden hunger, headaches, and crashes hit. Your tingling, cotton feet at the auction were one version of this.

For someone else, it might be falling asleep in front of the television after dinner or snapping at a spouse in the late afternoon. Another person might need a nap after an atypical lunch.

Food from boxes and cans adds more fuel. Boxed cereals and instant oats are often processed so heavily that they digest almost as fast as table sugar. Many so-called healthy cereals list "whole grain" on the front, but load sugar, syrups, and flavors just below it on the ingredient list.

Boxed rice and pasta mixes come with seasoning packets that combine refined starches, sugar, and flavor enhancers. Canned soups and sauces often contain added sugars alongside starches to create a thick, soothing texture and taste. The body is not dealing with the starch in the main food. It is also dealing with the hidden sugar in everything poured or sprinkled over it.

Restaurants lean on sugar for both taste and consistency. A sweet glaze helps meat brown and shine, and sugar stabilizes many sauces and dressings. Desserts are obvious sugar bombs. Items like sweet rolls, artisan breads, and certain sides are also tuned to hit the brain's reward centers.

The more the menu emphasizes house-made sauces and signature dressings, the more likely those recipes are to rely on sugar and refined starches as cheap crowd pleasers. Good-looking food is not pretty. It is tuned to keep your fork moving.

Doctors see the result of this pattern and give it names. Prediabetes, type 2 diabetes, metabolic syndrome, and fatty liver disease all grow more common with this way of eating. They warn about heart disease, stroke, kidney damage, nerve damage, and vision problems. They prescribe pills to push sugar down and tell people to lose weight and move more.

Often, they never ask what everyday food is made of. They hardly ever tally the bowls of cereal, sweet drinks, white flour, squeeze-bottle sauces, and ultra-processed snacks that train these bodies to spike, overreact, and then crash.

That morning at the auction is not drama for its own sake. It is a live picture of how close many people already are to the edge without knowing it. The more years people spend eating these foods, the less margin their bodies have.

For a twenty-five-year-old, a bowl of cereal might mean a quick sugar buzz and nothing more. At fifty-five or sixty-five, the same bowl can mean tingling feet and cotton steps. A pattern starts with small episodes at a produce auction and can end in constant numbness and a sense of being out of balance.

Sugar on a roller coaster never lives in its own box. It touches everything else this book has described. Ultra-processed foods that drive these spikes also carry emulsifiers, sprays, oxidized fats, and additives that inflame the gut, liver, and blood vessels. Each ride makes the body a little more fragile.

The more often we rely on boxed, canned, bottled, and restaurant food, the more danger we invite. These plates look normal, but keep pushing sugar and inflammation together.

Type 2 diabetes, heart disease, fatty liver, kidney trouble, stroke, depression, and sleep problems all appear more often in people who live on this pattern. Older people do not start waddling one morning by accident. Their joints, nerves, and vessels have been dealing with this roller coaster for decades, and the bill has at last come due.

The cereal bowl at the auction and the shiny plates at restaurants are part of the same story. It is not just too many carbs. It is a daily sugar carnival powered by processed grains, hidden sugars, and engineered taste.

Stepping off the ride is not about perfection or punishment. It is about giving nerves, eyes, kidneys, heart, and brain a chance to quiet down before the damage becomes permanent. In the next part, the focus shifts to what to do with this information. How to read menus, labels, and plates better, and how to spot sugar and starch traps before they slam into your bloodstream.

Chapter Eighteen

Tastes Great, Hurts Later

YOU SIT DOWN IN a busy restaurant, and everything feels right. Plates pass, piled with food that smells like comfort and looks just like the ads. You taste the first bite, and your brain lights up. Salt, fat, and a little sweet land in all the right places. This is not an accident.

Most restaurants are built to make food cheap, fast, and craveable, not to protect your long-term health. Behind most menus is the same wholesale machine. Restaurants do not stroll misty farms each morning, filling baskets by hand. They order from large distributors that also supply hospitals, nursing homes, stadiums, and chains.

The chicken breast or lettuce on your plate comes from the same system that fills grocery aisles, routed through another door. This is how the numbers work. Owners have to keep food costs low and tables full.

Bulk meat and poultry are often injected with brines and phosphates. Sauces come in buckets thickened, preserved, and sweetened to make cheap ingredients taste rich. Fryers are filled with industrial seed fats that can survive long hours at high heat, even as they oxidize and break down.

Restaurants have to pass the taste test, and they do. Sugar, salt, and fat are their tools. A little sugar slips into tomato sauce, slaw, and dressings, while soft white breads melt in your mouth because the fiber has been stripped away.

Squeezed sauces carry flavor, plus added sugars, gums, and natural flavors, which keep your brain asking for one more bite. Most owners don't think about their sugar or blood fats. They focus on food costs, reviews, and whether the Friday crowd will return.

If a sauce makes people order extra bread, it stays. If a sweet dressing keeps salads from coming back, it stays. There is no spreadsheet column for joint pain over the past 10 years. What happens after you leave your doctor's and your family's, not the line cook's?

The same wholesale system you have seen in earlier chapters dresses up when it walks into a dining room. Sprays cling to lettuce, tomatoes, grains, and oils. Modified corn and soy are used to make syrups, starches, and fats for sauces and breads.

Emulsifiers keep dressings and desserts smooth, while reheated seed fats feed inflammation and stress. The food looks appealing and passes the taste test, but it helps build heart disease, diabetes, fatty liver, kidney strain, and joint damage.

Most people already know pieces of this story. You have heard that fast food and junk food are not healthy, and that pesticides and additives are not your friends. What is new is seeing all the pieces in one picture.

When you realize the same system feeds restaurants, grocery stores, school cafeterias, stadiums, and your pantry, it becomes harder to dismiss pain as random bad luck. Being more conscious does not mean never eating out or avoiding menus forever.

It means that when a dish is good, cheap, and always the same, a small voice asks what was added to make it way. You start noticing that squeeze bottle sauces are not flavor but part of the chemical load your body must clear.

When restaurant plates become fuel several times a week, the risks of high blood pressure, sugar trouble, and joint pain climb, and they worsen with age. Most restaurant kitchens are not your mother's kitchen. They are small factories with better lights.

Owners care you enjoy tonight. What happens to you in ten years is someone else's department. Once you see it, you can still enjoy eating out without letting this wholesale, taste-first system run your life.

In the next chapter, the focus shifts from exposing the problem to moving through it. You will learn how to read menus clearly and choose less harmful dishes without becoming the difficult person at the table. You will see how to let restaurants be occasional entertainment rather than your primary fuel. That shift is where real leverage over your health begins.

Chapter Nineteen

Conclusion: Taking Your Kitchen Back

MOST RESTAURANT FOOD NOW acts like a slow poison. It looks normal, tastes excellent, and slowly wears down joints, vessels, nerves, and mood over the years. These systems are built to be cheap, craveable, and repeatable, not to keep your sugar steady or your brain clear.

The labels sit in warehouses, not on menus, so you seldom see the chemicals, broken oils, sugars, and factory meats on your plate. It is a magic show. The right hand flashes photos, sizzling pans, and smiling servers. The left hand stays hidden, running the machinery that turns cheap inputs into glossy food.

Stepping out of that spell does not mean never eating out again. It means no longer living as if the second kitchen were your only kitchen. One powerful, old-fashioned way to take control is to turn a patch of grass or patio space into a garden.

Even a few pots or small beds can grow lettuce, herbs, tomatoes, peppers, or beans you recognize at a glance. People who garden often eat more vegetables and fiber-rich foods, move more, and report less stress and a better mood. When you harvest your own food, its ingredient list lives in your memory, not on a package, because you watched it grow.

If you cannot grow much where you live, you can still buy smarter from people closer to the soil. Farmers' markets, produce stands, and local auctions often offer fresher fruits and vegetables than long-haul supermarket loads. Many small growers harvest at peak ripeness, so the food spends less time in storage and can hold more vitamins, minerals, and flavor.

Buying this way also gives you a clearer line of sight from field to plate. You may even find that some markets are cheaper for in-season produce than big stores. At Amish auctions in places like Ohio, much of the produce comes from small farms that rely more on soil care and tradition than on heavy processing.

You will have to find your own way to buy and eat better food. Everyone's life, money, and location are different. This book is not your new food Bible. Here is one way I do it.

I often drive into Amish areas and build genuine friendships there. Every couple of weeks, I stop at three to eight homes. I pull into driveways and see what they have.

Some days I come home with three to ten dozen eggs and two to ten pounds of butter. Other days I find vegetables, meat, chickens, rabbits, bacon, pork, honey, or whatever is in season. Sometimes a house has nothing that day. I thank them and move on to the next driveway.

I also visit Amish produce auctions and buy what I did not grow or could not grow. On the way home, I stop at a water place and fill twelve to twenty glass gallons for about twenty-five cents each. Some trips include a stop at an organic farmer-butcher for meat.

I know there is no perfect guarantee that no chemicals were ever used. But I see cows, pigs, and chickens moving in fields, and the eggs are fresh. I still buy some things at the grocery store, but I skip most boxed foods, canned goods, and frozen meals.

I pressure-can many foods when there is overflow. One year, I grew about two hundred pounds of potatoes and dry-pressure-canned them. That gave me forty quarts of potatoes for the next year, stored in glass without extra chemicals. I can turn those jars into mashed or scalloped potatoes in five minutes.

I started with simple water-bath canning about ten years ago and later moved into pressure canning for more foods. In some years, I put up as many as six hundred quarts. Some people rely on freezers, but we have had enough power outages that I trust glass jars more than a plug. Learning to store food in jars that can last for years, or to freeze-dry if you can, is another way to loosen the grip of the second kitchen.

I make time for this by watching less television and less news. I do the same with many vegetables and meats. My slow-cooked canned sausage is a favorite and disappears fast. Beets, beans, cabbage, and more go into jars. I have no grass in my backyard. It is all garden now.

Smart buying does not require perfection. It means asking a few quiet questions of your own choosing. How far did this travel? Who grew it? How many steps did it go through before it reached me?

When you can, you tilt your cart toward whole vegetables, fruits, beans, grains, eggs, and meats you can recognize. They may come from your yard, an Amish wagon, a market tent, or the better corner of a store. Each time you do, you starve the second kitchen a little and feed your own.

This is the invitation at the end of the story. Keep your eyes open at the magic show and learn to see the wires behind the trick. Let restaurants stay occasional entertainment, while your real fuel comes from food you can trace from soil to plate.

Turning even a small patch of yard into herbs and vegetables is one way to start turning down the poison. Visiting local growers when you can adds to that effort. Cooking a few more meals at home each week strengthens it further.

Every simple meal you grow or choose with care is a vote for clearer joints, steadier sugar, and a calmer mind. It is also a vote for a life where your own kitchen, not the second one, has the last word.

Chapter Twenty

Bibliography

American Medical Association. "What Doctors Wish Patients Knew About Ultraprocessed Foods." 2025.

Chassaing, B., et al. "Food Emulsifiers and Metabolic Syndrome: The Role of the Gut Microbiota." 2022.

Harvard T. H. Chan School of Public Health. "Food Additives and Health."

Healthline. "Are Pesticides in Foods Harming Your Health" 2017.

Johns Hopkins Bloomberg School of Public Health. "Ultraprocessed Foods Account for More Than Half of Calories Consumed at Home." 2024.

Kelly, J. R., et al. "Food Additive Emulsifiers and Their Impact on Gut Microbiome, Gut Barrier and Host Metabolism." *Journal of Crohn's and Colitis*, 2021.

Lane, M. M., et al. "Ultra-Processed Food Exposure and Adverse Health Outcomes: Umbrella Review of Observational Studies." *BMJ*, 384:e077310, 2024.

Martino, C., et al. "The Key to Intestinal Health: A Review and Perspective on Food Additives." 2024.

National Heart, Lung, and Blood Institute / National Institutes of Health. "Spotlight on UPFs: NIH Explores Link Between Ultraprocessed Foods and Heart Disease." 2025.

National Institutes of Health / National Center for Biotechnology Information. "Ultra-Processed Foods: What They Are and How to Identify Them."

Nature Communications. "Common Dietary Emulsifiers Promote Metabolic Disorders and Gut Inflammation." 2024.

NPIC (National Pesticide Information Center, Oregon State University). "Older Adults and Pesticides: Fact She et."

Stanford Medicine. "Ultra-Processed Food: Five Things to Know." 2025.

U.S. Department of Health and Human Services, Food and Drug Administration, and U.S. Department of Agriculture. "Address the Health Risks of Ultra-Processed Foods." 2025.

Vovk, Marko. *How to Start Writing*. Draft booklet, 2025.

Vovk, Marko. *Poisoned at the Grocery Store: Why Shopping Fresh Is Not Enough to Escape a Toxic Food Supply*. FixYourToxicHome.com, 2025.

World Cancer Research Fund. "Ultra-Processed Foods Linked to Increased Cancer Risk, Diabetes, and Heart Disease." 2025.

World Health Organization. "Pesticide Residues in Food." 2022.

Yale Medicine. "Are Ultraprocessed Foods Bad for Your Health" 2025.

Yale School of Public Health. "Ultra-Processed Foods Information Sheet." 2025.

Ultra-Processed Foods and Human Health. The Lancet Series, 2025.

"Pesticide Exposure, Associated Risks, and Chronic Disease." Systematic review, 2024.

"Hidden Dangers in Food and Environment: Pesticides and Gut Health." IPA Biotics, 2025.

Chapter Twenty-One

Further Reading by Marko Vovk

Main Collection

BIAS: How Our Minds Deceive Us – 18 Ways Your Perceptions Are Skewed and How to See More Clearly

Childless Cat Lady – Movement, Dynamics, Health, and Political Influence

Don't Rent This Home, Condo, or Apartment

Empty Cradles – Declining Birth Rates Explained

Fix Your Toxic Home and Live Longer

Forever Chemicals – How PFAS Pollutes Our Blood and Lives

Make Your Home Great Again (For Homeowners and Buyers) – Expanded Tips Edition

Nuclear Extinction Event Is Killing Our Families

Pets: The Hidden Costs of Companionship

Poisoned at the Grocery Store – Why Shopping Fresh Is Not Enough to Escape a Toxic Food Supply

Project 2025 Quick Review

Surviving Electrosmog – How to Understand and Reduce

Invisible Pollution in Your Home and Life
The Sixth Extinction: Return to Earth 2225 – Dystopian fiction about how the Anunnaki return to a scarred Earth with only 500,000 people left.
Heaven Is a Misfiled Ticket – A comic novel about a man who is sent to the wrong heavens by mistake.
The Water You Drink May Be Killing You
No-Mow Living – The Real Hidden Costs of Grass

Forthcoming Books (2026–2027)

(Working titles; final names may change)
Pressure Canning: Preservation of Food
Above-Ground Gardening
Grow Your Own Teas – How to Harvest and Blend Them for Holistic Use
Trump's First Year – A Highly Political Review
The Concrete Dressed-Up Duck – A reality-fiction novel about a yard duck that quietly watches the houses across the street (Spring 2026)

Many of these longer works will also be adapted into shorter guides and papers in 2026–2027.

White Papers

Hidden Drivers of Population Decline – How Modern Health, Environmental, and Medical Risks Create Empty

Cradles
Indoor Pets, Hidden Costs – Health, Housing, Money, and the Environment in Pet-Centric Living

Earth Helpers Kids' Series

PFAS KIDS – The Forever Chemical Mystery
The Great Smoke, Fire & Dust Adventure
EMF KIDS – The Secret World of Invisible Waves
Nuclear KIDS – Little Lessons from Atomic Power
Grass KIDS – Why the Lawn Isn't Always Greener
Home Safety KIDS – Smart Habits for Everyday Dangers
Lucky to Be Alive – Discover Why Every Life Is a Miracle
The Vitamin ABC's – A Healthy Kids' Guide

Eight additional Earth Helpers Kids' Series titles are planned for 2026–2027.
To find any of these titles, search for "Marko Vovk" on Amazon.

Made in the USA
Monee, IL
04 November 2026

67381918R00066